SMOKEBREAKER

A 90 day guide to free you from cigarettes forever.

PAUL F BARRY

Smokebreaker
Copyright © 2019 by Paul F Barry

All rights reserved. No part of this publication may be reproduced, distributed, or transmitted in any form or by any means, including photocopying, recording, or other electronic or mechanical methods, without the prior written permission of the author, except in the case of brief quotations embodied in critical reviews and certain other non-commercial uses permitted by copyright law.

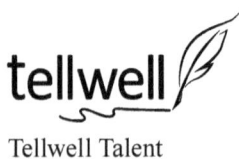

Tellwell Talent
www.tellwell.ca

ISBN
978-0-2288-1946-2 (Paperback)

Smokebreaker™

No Withdrawal!
No Drugs!
Smoke like always 'til you quit!

A Testimonial

This is the story of a guy who smoked a pack of cigarettes a day from the time he was sixteen 'til the time he quit at the age of forty-three.

I liked to smoke. It was as simple as that. I also grew up at a time when smoking was promoted on TV... by doctors, for heaven's sake! It was not only cool... it was 'good' for you... or at least that was what the advertising implied. In this atmosphere, I never tried to quit and was never given any incentive to do so.

As time went by, the world's attitude toward smoking changed. We discovered that it really wasn't all that good for you. In fact, we discovered that it could... and would harm you. So began the many failed attempts to quit. Every once in a while, I said to myself, "OK, I guess I should!" and would try to stop. That usually lasted for less than a day. If I was really serious, I could make it into the next day. When, on occasion, I stopped for a couple of days, my secretary would go out and buy me a pack of cigarettes because she couldn't stand my 'edginess.' That's a nice way of saying that I became a big pain in the @$$!

What finally made up my mind to quit permanently was a news item that stated, 'Even if you had smoked as much as two packs a day and were under forty-five years of age, and did quit, in seven years it would be as though you had never smoked.' That was the push I needed.

After mapping out a strategy, I started my program.

<u>NINETY DAYS LATER... I QUIT... FOR GOOD!!</u> ... and with no withdrawal symptoms!!

That was many years ago... and I have never smoked since... nor have I wanted to! I'm thrilled to share this program with you now. I promise that if you strictly adhere to the program, YOU WILL QUIT TOO!!

Now, it's time for you to meet my special team and begin your journey.

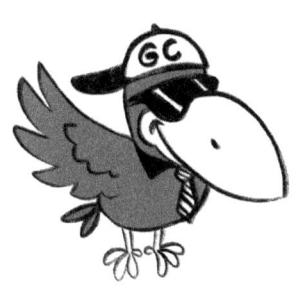

Hi...I'm Crow Naggin', Man. I'll be your GC (that's Guardian Crow) for the next ninety days. I'm gonna help you get thru' this program... I promise!

The journey on which you are about to embark requires no sacrifice or discomfort on your part. I do, however, demand one thing.

You must follow the instructions exactly. Let me repeat that. **<u>YOU MUST FOLLOW THE INSTRUCTIONS EXACTLY!!</u>**

That won't be hard... but make no mistake: this is not a 'maybe I will and maybe I won't today' program. If you stray from the program at any time…

<u>YOU MUST START ALL OVER... FROM THE BEGINNING!</u> Straying will mean adding to the total time quitting will take.

I guarantee, however, that if you follow the instructions that we lay out in your book…

<u>YOU WILL STOP SMOKING!!</u> ...and you won't be cranky! And you won't kick your dog! ...and your friends won't avoid you!

OK. Ready for your journey? Let's begin.

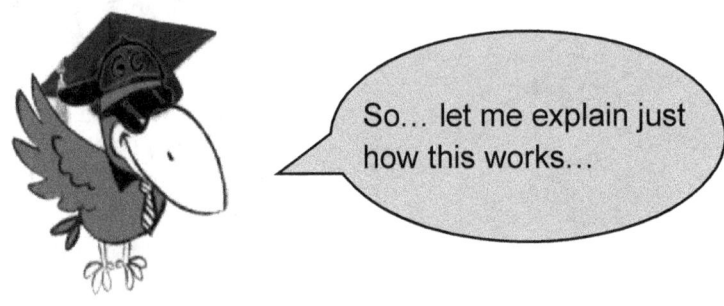

...we're talkin' about (this is where I get scientific. Ready?)

...positive, self-focused brainwashing.

Right! I said... **brainwashing!**
Only this is good brainwashing.
And to make it work, you gotta be...

1.) **Enthused about your new commitment; and you gotta...**
2.) **Repeat this to yourself, OUT LOUD... hundreds of times... and you gotta**
3.) **Say it like you mean it.**

After all, this is a good thing you're doing, and now, you will expect good things to happen!

See how simple this is?

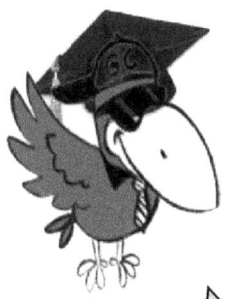

To make it easy to track your progress, why not start on a Monday...

And why don't you mark the final day on a calendar. That way you'll have a definite 'quit day.'

OK? Let's get started!

Remember how the cover of your book says… "Smoke like always 'til you quit"?

Well, we mean it. The only thing you will do differently is…

BEFORE EACH CIGARETTE, YOU MUST REPEAT THE DAY'S MANTRA!

Day 1

Mantra

Remember… say this before every cigarette!

(You don't have to say it out loud if you don't want to, but it's better if you do.)

I've got to keep smoking for another eighty-nine days. As much as I hate smoking, I'll keep at it until it's time to quit.

Day 2

Mantra

Oh man... I've gotta keep smoking for another eighty-eight days.

What a drag!

I hate these things, but I did promise to keep smoking like always.

Day 3

Mantra

Gee, I hate smoking. And it is annoying having to say this every time I light up.

I'm starting to hate everything about smoking!

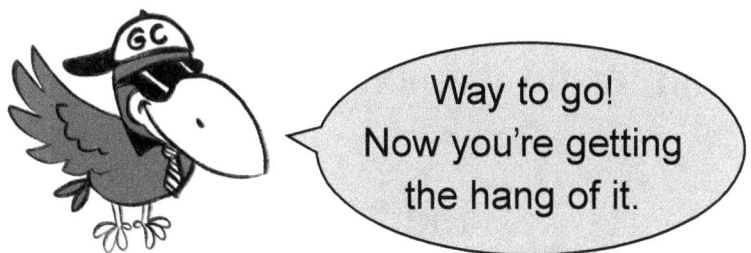

Day 4

Mantra

Wow, still eighty-six days to go… but I won't quit yet.

I'll smoke every day like always 'til the end of the program… no matter how much I hate smoking.

And I do!!!!

Day 5

Mantra

I'm gonna keep smoking, every day… no matter how much I hate this.

I promised I would keep smoking, but I'd like to quit…

NOW!!

Day 6

Mantra

(People think I'm nuts, talking to myself every time I light up. But I don't care. When this is all over, they'll understand.) In the meantime,

I am another day closer to being able to quit these awful things.

I can do this.

Day 7

Mantra

Hey! First week down...
Only twelve weeks to go!!

Boy, I hate this! I've gotta keep smoking for another twelve weeks... eighty-three more days!! AAAAAHHHGGGG!

Day 8

Start of a brand-new week. Keep it up... you're doing great!

Mantra

You know, I really don't like smoking, but I've got to keep at it... for the next eighty-two days.

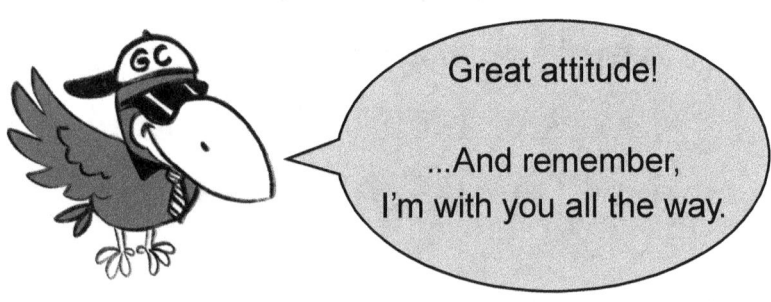

Day 9

Mantra

It'll be so great when I can finally quit!

Think of all the money I'm going to save. But I can't quit yet…

No matter how much I hate it, I'm going to keep going!

Day 10

Mantra

Still a long way to go.

These things are starting to taste bad… Gee, I really do hate smoking.

But in only eighty days, I can quit!

But not yet...

Day 11

Mantra

I'm just realizing how much time I waste just smoking!

Wish I could quit right now... but I'll keep going for another seventy-nine days!!! YIKES!!!

Day 12

Mantra

I'm starting to dread every time I pull out a cigarette.

Wow, do I ever hate these things.

Day 13

Mantra

Every day that goes by brings me closer to the day I can quit!

I can hardly wait.

In the meantime, I've gotta keep smoking!
…and I hate it!

Day 14

Mantra

Sometimes I feel I'm all alone, but GC says he's always around. Hope so!

Hey, another week down, number two. This is really starting to get to me. I really hate these darn cigarettes. I want to quit but I can't yet… Only another seventy-six days to go.

Day 15

Mantra

You know, I really believe that I hate these things.

I know I'll be able to quit now.

Hey, look who's back!

Hi GC!

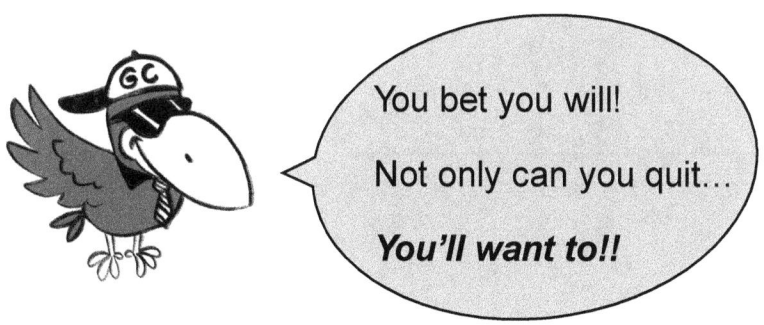

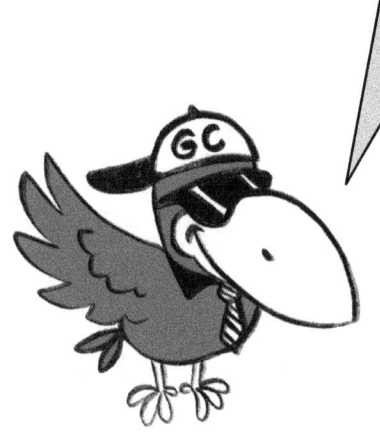

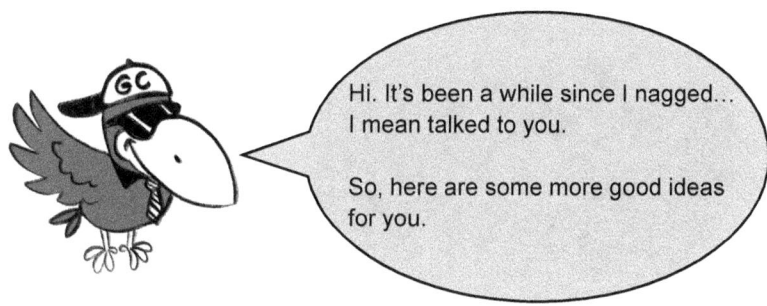

Today, I'm offering some thoughts that may give you even more reasons to quit. Notice I didn't say 'more reasons to **_want_** to quit.' I figure you already really want to, so these are just things you might not have put down on paper yet.

OK, let's talk cost!!

Boy oh boy, is this ever one to ponder.

If you are anything like my alter ego was when he smoked, you're probably going through at least a pack a day. BTW, he was smoking a pack and a half a day. This was back in the days of $1.75 a pack, so it was costing him approximately $80 a month.

Last time I checked, a pack cost anywhere from $8 to $12. Holy cow, that's as much as $540 a month or, wait for it… $6,480.00 a year. Yikes.

Think about this. If you saved that amount for the next three years, you'd have nearly $20,000.00 in the bank.

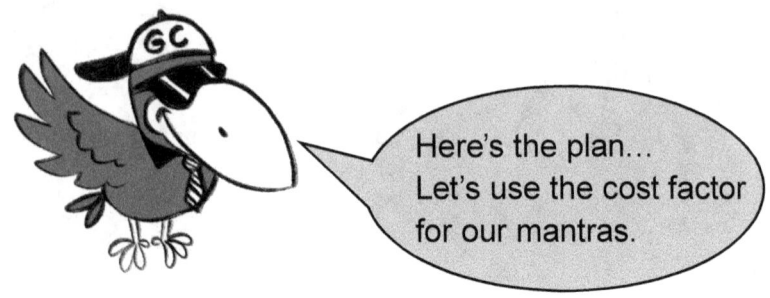

Ohm…. (I heard this in a Pilates class once)

Mantra

In three years, I can save enough in the bank to buy a newer car and I won't have to scrimp or change my routine at all.

What a good idea.

Thanks, GC.

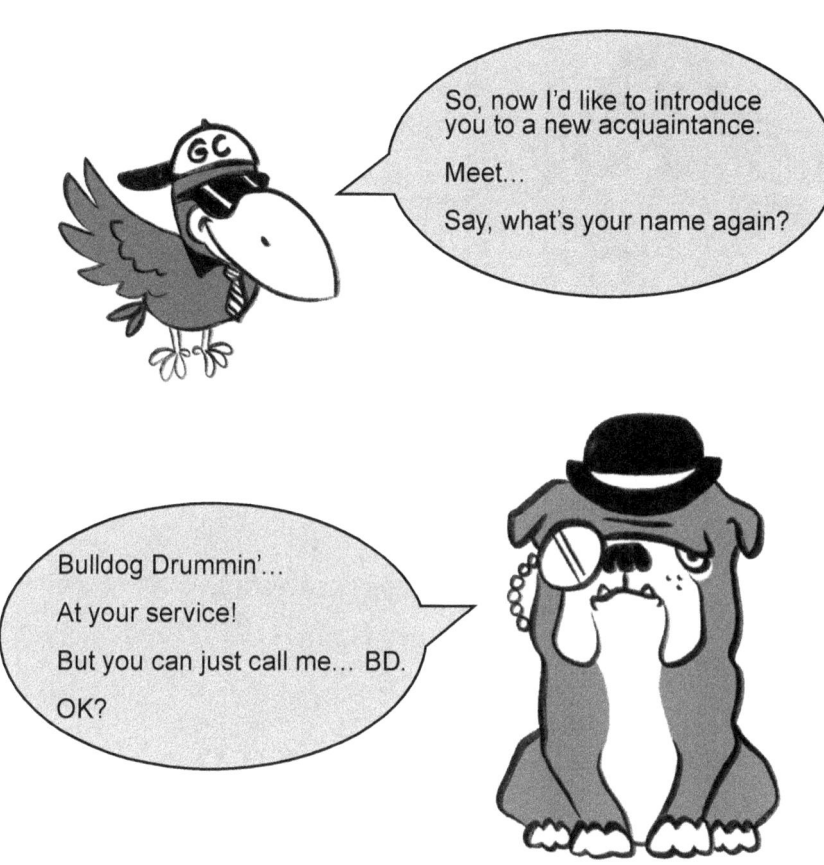

"Hey, didn't you used to be a famous detective?"

"Naw, that was another guy. I'm called a 'reinforcer'… I remind people about any task they've taken on and help them to stay on track. I just look tough… but I'm really a nice guy and a bit of a softy. Hope I can be of help on your journey."

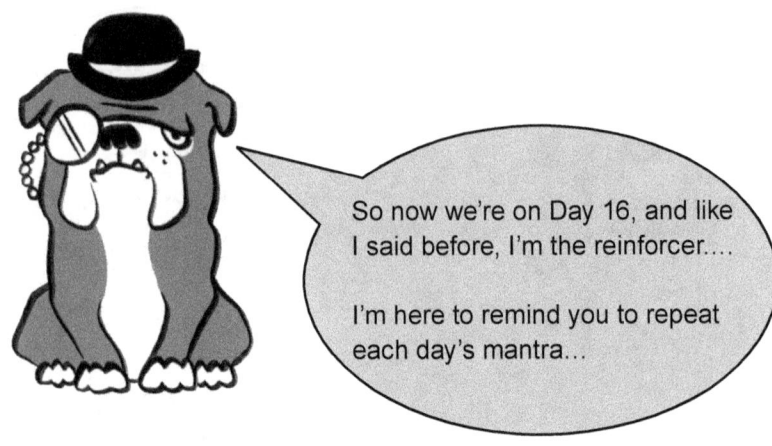

Seriously now…
To make this program work,
(watch my lips),

REPEAT THE MANTRA… OUT LOUD!!!

In three years, I can have enough in the bank to buy a newer car and I won't have to scrimp or change my routine at all.
…and don't forget to say this before every cigarette!

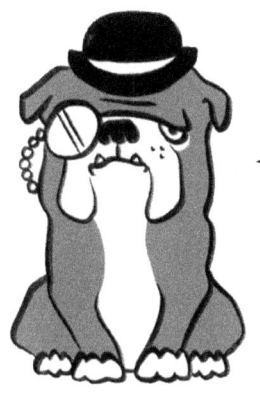

Now you've got it! Way to go.

Hey, I'm going to stick around for a week or so while our pal GC takes a break.

So here goes…

Day 17

Mantra

This is great. I can save over six grand a year now. So, what can I do with that? A cruise through the Caribbean! That'd be nice.

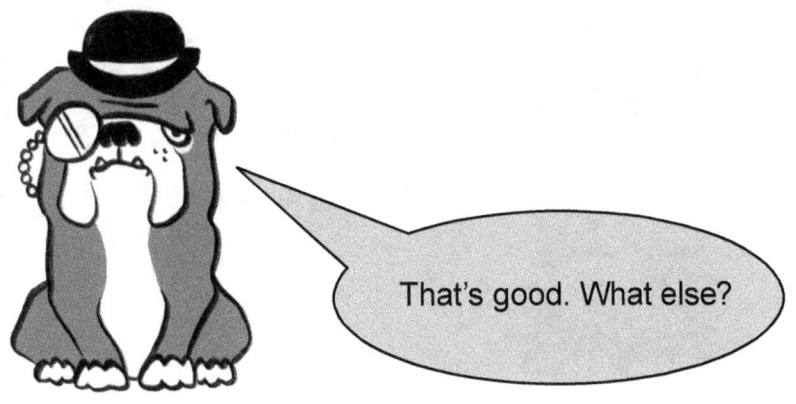

Day 18

Now, think about what else you'd like to have.

Mantra

I can buy a whole new wardrobe with what I'll be saving.

Day 19

Mantra

I really hate these things, but I promised I wouldn't quit for ninety days. Only seventy-one days to go. I can do this!

Day 20

Mantra

I keep thinking about all that money I'm going have…

I can take a cruise *and* get a new wardrobe!

Ooh, I'm liking this idea.

Day 21

Hey, it's been three weeks already! This isn't as easy as I thought, though.

Mantra

I can't quit smoking yet, but I hate these #*^# cigs... and I can't wait to quit!!

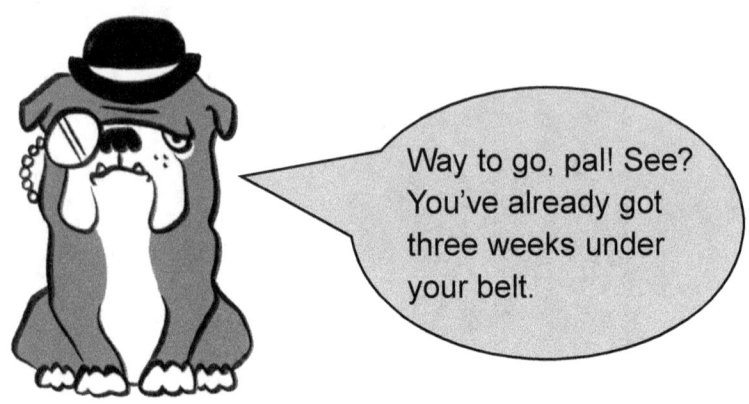

**You should be proud of yourself.
This is a good milestone.
Less than ten weeks to go.**

**I promise you …
If you do as GC and I say…**

YOU'RE GONNA MAKE IT!

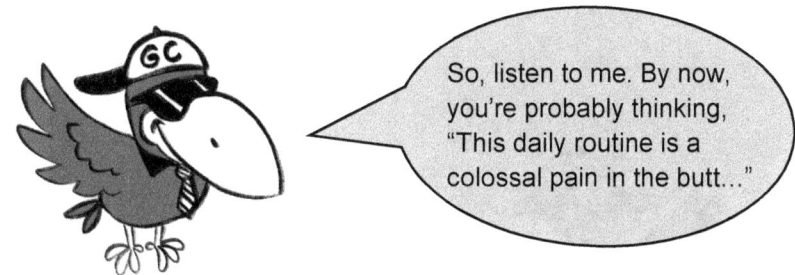

"Well, it's supposed to be! That's how this whole program works, right, BD?"

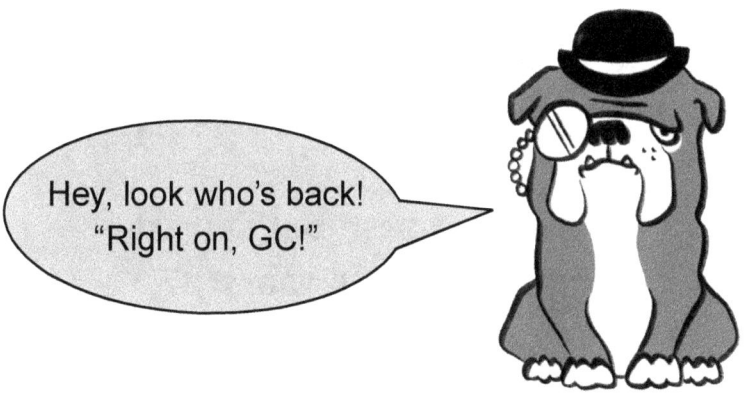

"And let me reinforce (remember, that's what I do) your task.

Every day, with every cigarette, you must repeat the day's mantra. Don't kid yourself… if you don't, this whole program won't work. And like GC said at the beginning of your journey… if you even skip one day = you'll have to start all over again."

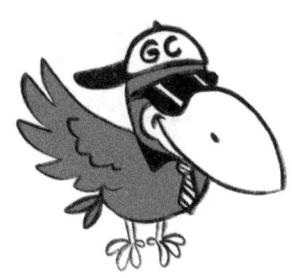 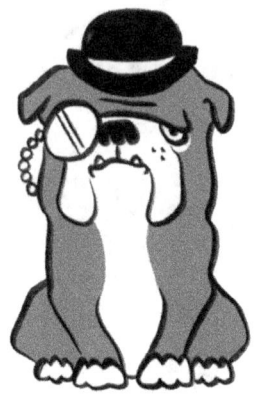

"Please, please! From both of us... <u>*repeat the day's mantra every time you light up!*</u>

Out loud is best, but at least
do it silently to yourself.

OK, this is as good a time as
any... and be honest:
are you doing this every time you light up?

Look, missing a couple of times is
OK, but if you're not doing it, this is a
perfect time to back to page one and...

START OVER!!!!"

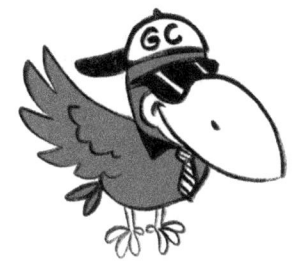

Think about what we're doing here. We want you to be p'....d off!

We only told you that this would be easy. We didn't say you'd like it. In fact, that's the whole idea! Soon… and then forever, you'll be associating cigarettes with a feeling of disgust, annoyance, and just downright "peed-off-ness!" Hey BD, I just coined a new word.

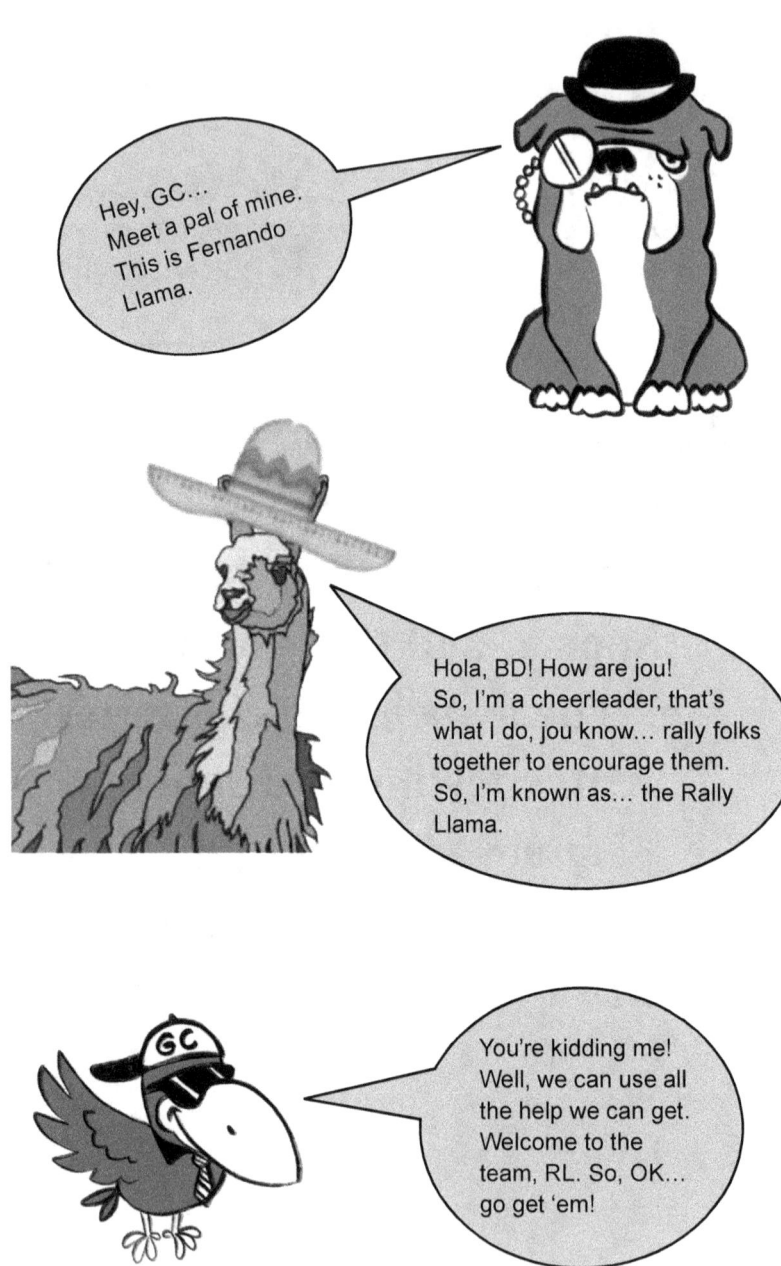

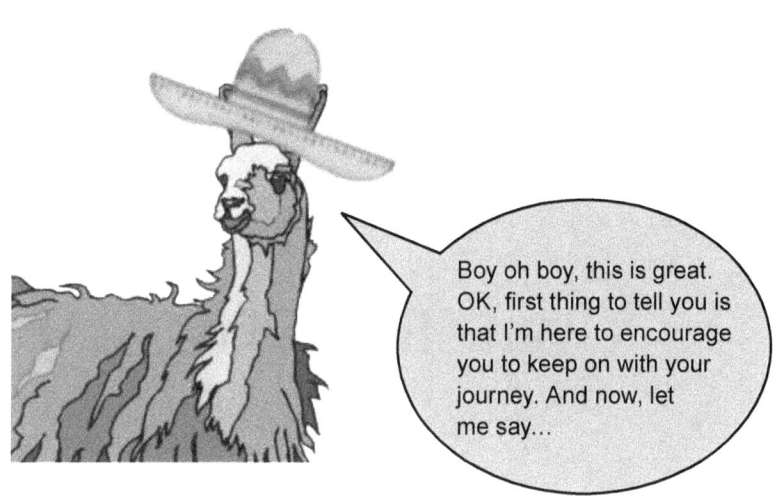

...Jou look mawrvelous! Jou really do! And jou should be proud of what jou're doing. Jou're already into three weeks now, and youst think: only nine weeks to go. I'll be here to cheer jou on at every step, so here we go... Today's Mantra is back to basics!

As much as I hate these things, I gotta keep smoking for another nine weeks.

Then finally I can quit! I can hardly wait.

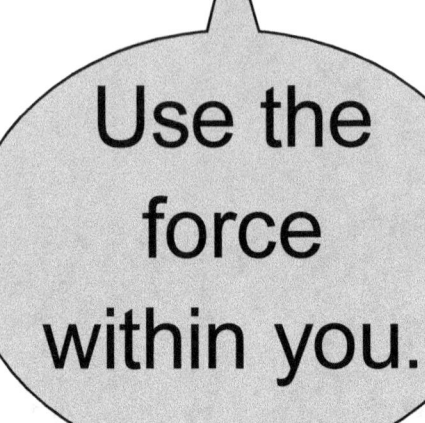
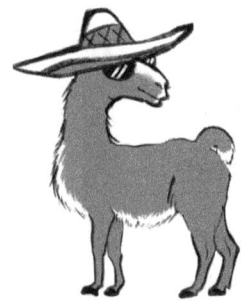
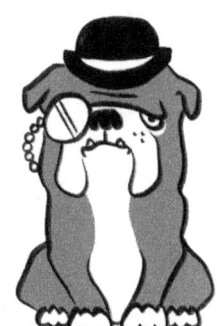
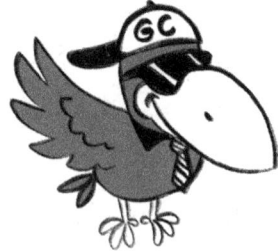

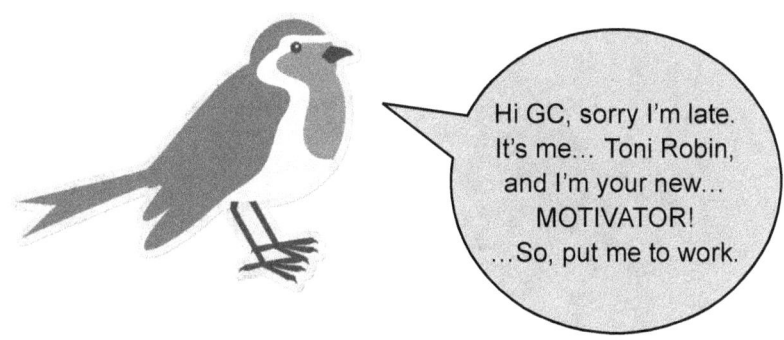

GC tells me you're already starting on week four. Boy, that's great. OK, so here we go!

Mantra

Oh, I hate these #%@& cigarettes!

But I will keep smoking them every day like always. Can't quit yet.

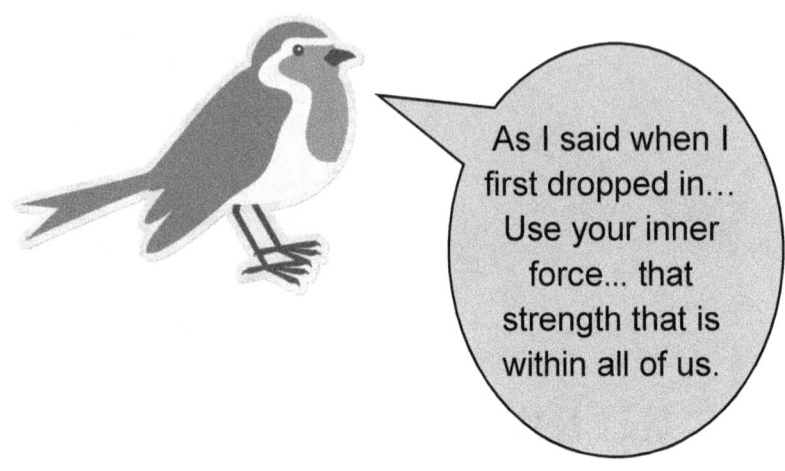

Mantra

I'm really starting to dislike everything about cigarettes.

They leave a bad taste in my mouth and give me a slight headache all the time.

Day 22

Mantra

I'm really looking forward to finally being able to quit these things.

Day 23

Mantra

Another day and I gotta keep
smoking these dumb cigarettes.
I promised I wouldn't
quit for ninety days.

Day 24

Mantra

This is not a lot of fun!

...But I really do hate these rotten cigarettes!

Day 25

Mantra

Oh, how I wish I could quit today!

But I've gotta keep smoking
for another five weeks.

Day 26

Mantra

This isn't so hard... just annoying!

I hate these foul-tasting cigarettes!

Day 27

Mantra

Another week out of the way!

Only five more to go… Can't quit yet, but I'd sure like to!

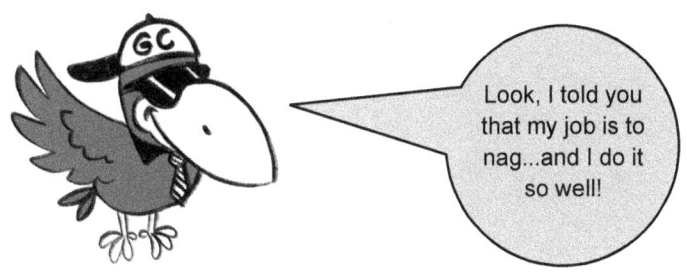

...but I don't want to be in your face every day. And I don't think it's necessary either 'cause you're doing so well.

So, for the next four weeks, one of us will check in with you on the weekend. Oh, you'll have a daily mantra for sure, but we're going to rely on your commitment to this program. All you'll need to do is… REPEAT THE DAILY MANTRA… EVERY TIME YOU LIGHT UP! How's that for a final nag! See you in a week.

Day 28

Reminder:

You must smoke as much as you always do. Don't cut back... even if you want to!

Mantra

I've got another sixty-two days to keep up this disgusting habit… Can't quit yet, but I can hardly wait 'til I can.

Day 29

Mantra

One day at a time…

Wow, I really hate these things.

Day 30

Mantra

I wish I could quit today, but I promised to keep on smoking 'til the end of the program.

But I hate these things!!

Day 31

Mantra

These things make me feel awful… Makes me wonder why I ever started. I want to quit, but I've got another fifty-nine days to go.

Day 32

Mantra

I'm ready to quit,
but I know all the gang will be
on my case if I try to quit now.

Ok, here goes another one.

Day 33

Mantra

These things really do taste awful, and now I'm noticing just how messy they are.

Day 34

Mantra

As much as I hate these things, I will keep smoking 'til the program ends. After all, I did promise!

Day 35

Mantra

Oh boy! End of week five.

Looks like I'm making some progress, 'cause I really do hate these things!

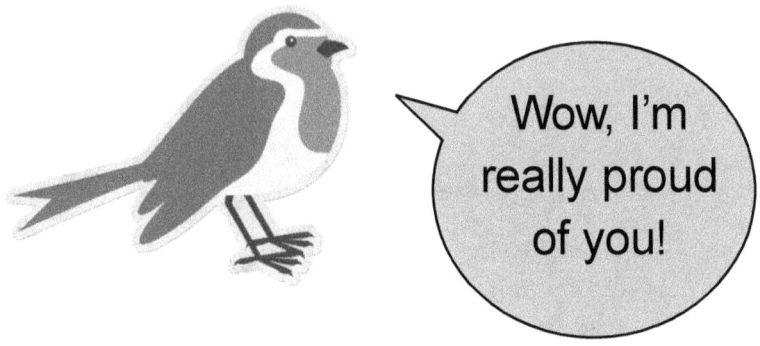

Just look at how far you've come…
You're almost halfway there.
Only another eight weeks and you'll
be free of this terrible addiction.

Keep up the good work, and I'll
see you in a couple of weeks when
you're on the home stretch.
Cheers!

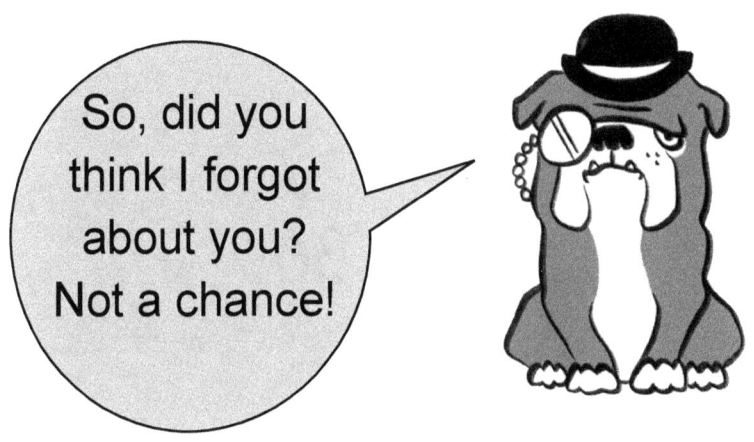

Remember, I'm the reinforcer.
So now... and I want you to be honest with me (and more importantly, yourself), have you been repeating the daily mantra out loud... before each time you light up?

You know that's the only way this is going to work. If you have, 'good on you!'

Please keep at it, just like we talked about, and… **<u>You will succeed</u>**! I promise! OK, let's begin week six... Go get 'em!

Day 36

Mantra

Note to self:

When I quit, I'm going to save the amount I've been spending on these stupid cigarettes.

I can save up to $6500 a year. Wow, I can hardly wait to quit.

Day 37

Mantra

When I quit smoking these awful things, think about all the things I'll be able to do with all that money I'll be saving… could be as much as $20,000. Wow!!

Only eight weeks to go!

Day 38

Mantra

What a drag... these cigs are driving me crazy, and I hate 'em.

Day 39

Mantra

As soon as I quit, I know
I'll start to feel better.
When I think about it, this is
the best idea I've ever had.
There's no downside.

Day 40

Mantra

Jumpin' Nellie,
I really hate these things.

Maybe I could cut back...

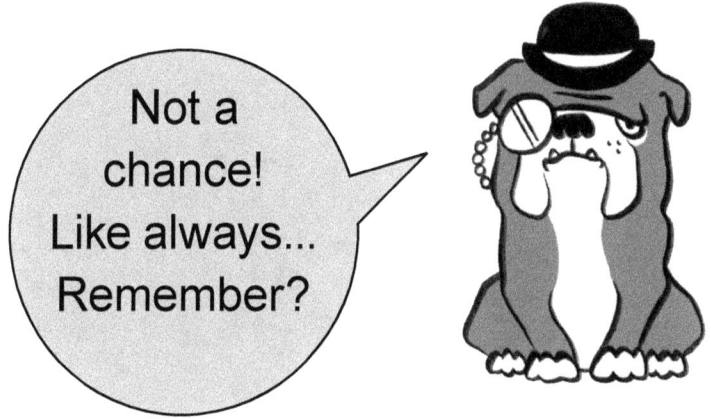

Just to let you know, I'm still here,
just not 'in your face' so much.

I know you want to quit,
but we all agreed…
You've got to keep smoking
like you always did no matter
how much you hate it. That's
the whole point, isn't it?

Day 41

Mantra

Thanks, BD!

I appreciate your being here.

Okay. I'll keep on smoking these awful things even tho' I really hate them.

Day 42

Mantra

Hey, it's the end of another week.
Gettin' to the halfway point.
But oh, how I hate these things.

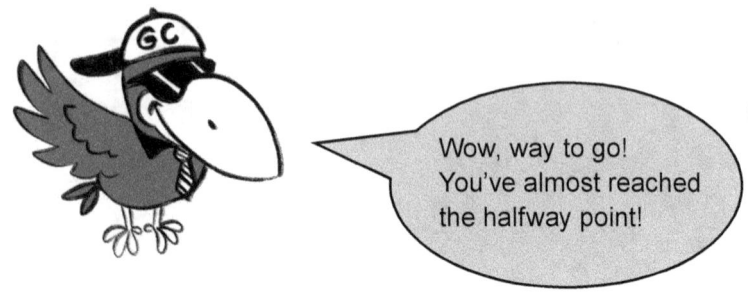

My whole team is really proud of you.

We're on the home stretch now.

Another forty-five days and a bit and you can start enjoying a whole new life.

Keep up the good work.

I think it's time for Toni Robin to do her thing.

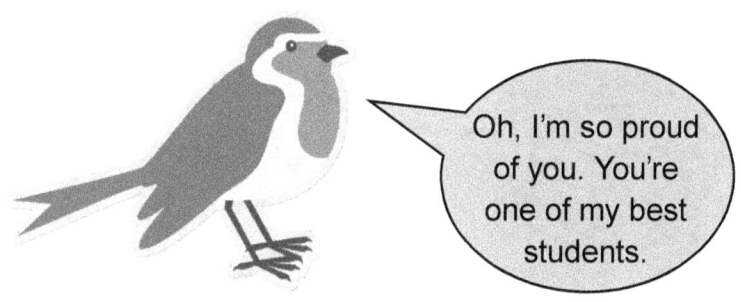

From what I've seen and heard… you are doing a great job by yourself.
That's because you've tapped that 'inner force' I spoke about earlier. You may be surprised that you are doing this by yourself... but I'm not.

I knew you could do it all along. Way to go! Now on to the second half.

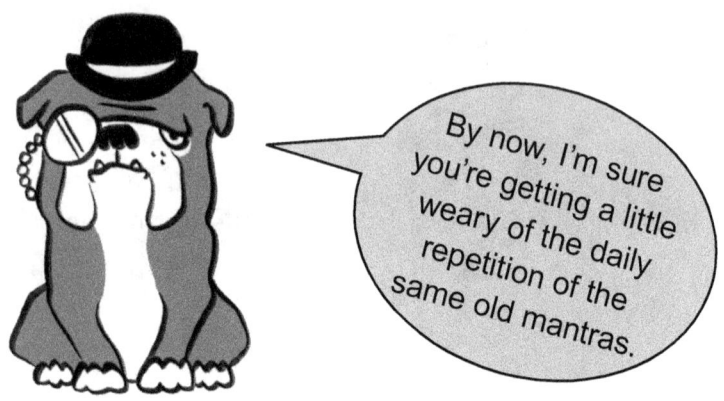

It probably seems boring, and

maybe you've thought that you
don't really need to repeat them
every time you light up.

Let me assure you… (remember,
I'm the reinforcer)…
It's important, no, ***IT'S VITAL***,
that you repeat the mantras
every time you light up.

This program only works if you do.

You've come too far to have to
start all over again. Right?

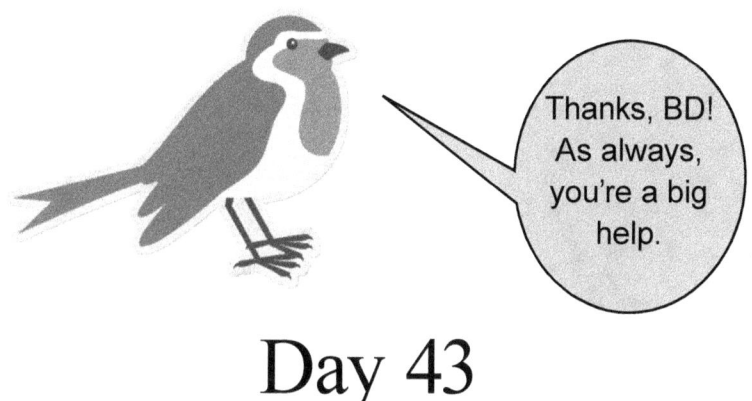

Day 43

Okay, let's get moving.

Today's Mantra

Wow, I've gotta keep smoking
for another forty-seven days.
...And I hate these awful cigarettes.

Day 44

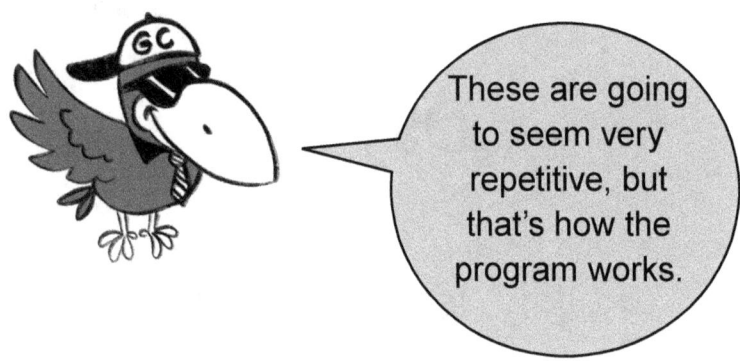

Mantra

I really hate smoking now. These cigarettes are really starting to taste awful.

Day 45

Mantra

Another day and I must keep smoking. I'd really like to quit now, but I gotta keep going for another forty-five days.

Hey, I'm halfway there already.

Day 46

Mantra

Wow, I'm on the home stretch!
Only seven weeks to go…
I can do this.
I will keep smoking like always,
but… I really hate these things.

Day 47

Mantra

I've been smoking for a long time…
I guess I've just been
doing it out of habit.

It really is a waste of
time and money…
I can't wait to quit!

Day 48

Mantra

Give me strength! I hate these things.

Day 49

Mantra

Great, here's another week gone by! Getting closer to my "Quit Day"… If only I could quit right now.

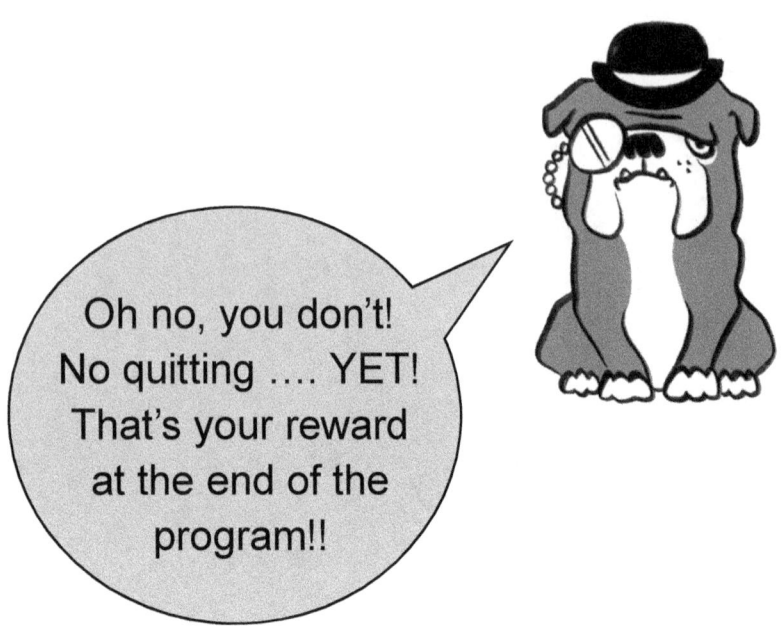

I'm going to get RL to jump in now and take over for a while. You ready, RL?

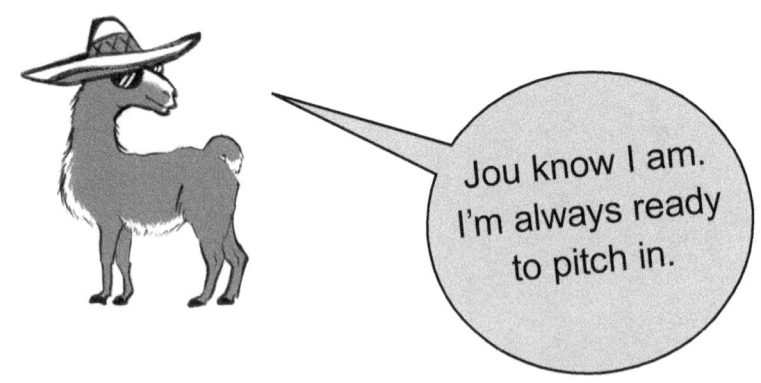

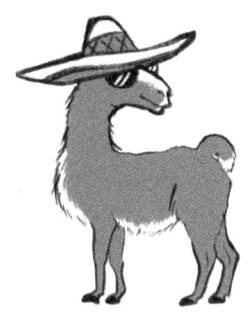

> I've missed jou! So, let's get going again... And by the way... can I say... Jou look mahvelous!! Jes jou do!

So, here we are at the start of another week. ...and I'm so proud of jou. Jou've come through seven weeks of the program and jou're going to make it. I promise! Now I'll get out of jour face and let jou concentrate on each of the next seven days.

Day 50

Mantra

(This is going to be harder because jou're really starting to hate these awful cigarettes.)

Gotta keep smoking as much as I ever did. Can't quit now, even though I want to.

Day 51

Mantra

I'm also getting tired of having to repeat these stupid mantras every time I light up.

I hate smoking so much, but I'll be able to quit soon.

Day 52

Mantra

I think I'm getting a constant headache from all this smoking. Smoking sure doesn't seem as enjoyable as it was before. After I quit, I'll feel much better.

Day 53

Mantra

How great it will be when I can finally stop smoking these awful and expensive cigarettes.

Day 54

Mantra

Only a few more weeks to go… and then I can finally quit these things. I gotta stay with it, now.

Day 55

Mantra

This is getting to be a drag.
I hate these awful cigarettes.

Day 56

Mantra

Wow!! Another week down. Getting closer to the big day when I CAN QUIT!!!

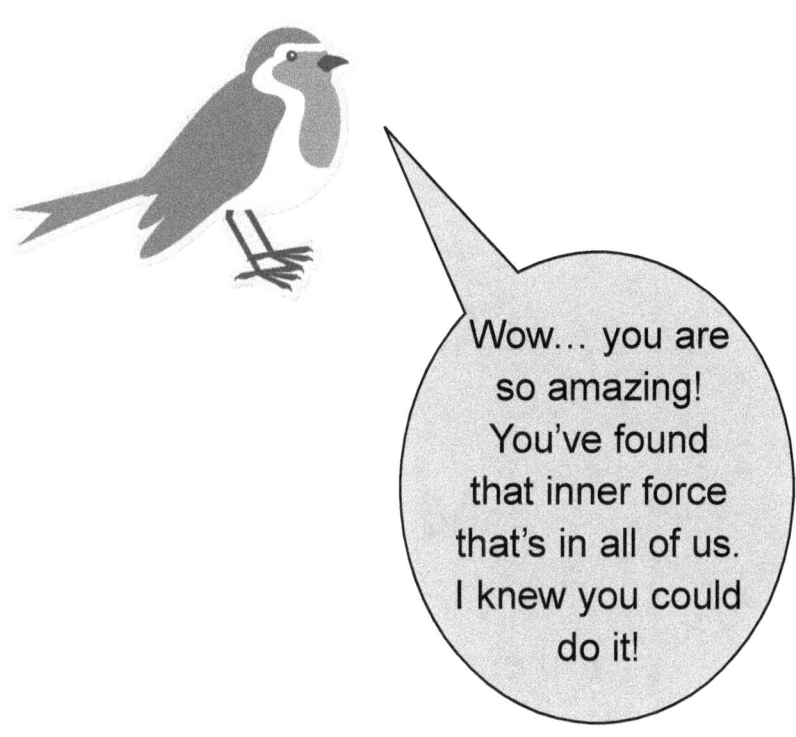

Now reach deep down
and let it guide you over
the next five weeks…

Together we're going to reach
the finish line when you can rid
yourself of this terrible addiction.
OK! Here we go…

Day 57

Mantra

Another day of these awful cigarettes. I'm not a quitter, so I've gotta keep smoking.

(That's funny... I gotta keep smoking so I can quit!)

Day 58

Mantra

I'll be so happy when I won't have to do this every day.

Day 59

Mantra

I hate this horrible habit.
I wish I'd never started
in the first place!

Day 60

Mantra

In fewer than five weeks, I'll be free of these things…

Day 61

Mantra

I can't wait to start feeling better…
No headaches,
and I'm told that
food will taste better.

Day 62

Mantra

Wow, it's the weekend already. Starting week ten in two days. I can do this.

Day 62

Mantra

I don't care if people think I'm nuts… I'm gonna beat these things.

Day 63

Mantra

Another week down!!
Boy, I hate these things!!
But I will keep at it.

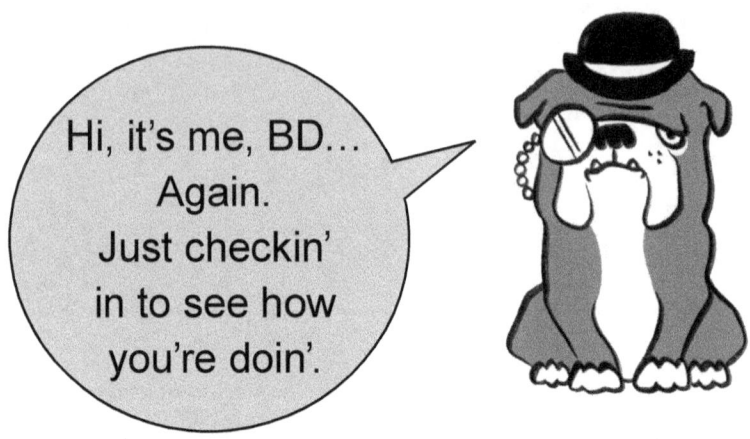

Hi, it's me, BD… Again. Just checkin' in to see how you're doin'.

I know I can be a pain sometimes, but I'm just doin' my job.

I am the reinforcer, after all.

If you've been honest with yourself and you've been repeating the daily mantras as I hope you have, you've just about beaten the odds and gotten closer to your goal of quitting.

Keep it up, and remember: we're all pulling for you.

Day 64

Mantra

Only four weeks to go...
one more month!

Gotta keep smoking... every day.
Boy, do I ever hate these things.

Day 65

Mantra

This is getting to be a real pain!
I want to quit now…
But I promised I'd keep smoking every day for another four weeks.

Day 66

Mantra

(Must repeat the daily mantra every time I light up.)

Can't quit yet…

But I do hate these things.

Day 67

Mantra

These things stink... and I know I make a mess every time I butt out. I hate smoking!!!

Day 68

Mantra

In less than four weeks, I'll be free of all this mess and hassle.

Won't that be great!

Day 69

Mantra

Oh boy, just about got another week behind me. Wish I could quit now.

Day 70

Mantra

Wonder if it's ok to quit now.
This program is a real
pain in the neck.
...and I've only got three
more weeks to go.

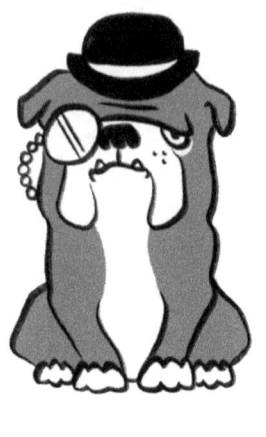

Oh no you don't! Did you think I'd let you off this easily? Remember, I'm here to help you get through this ordeal.

You're doing so great and I knew you'd be one of my best charges.

I'm right here to keep you focused on the goal…

You will quit … in just three more weeks. So stay with me, OK?

Day 71

Thanks, BD! I needed that. Ok, just three more weeks to go.

Mantra

I can do this…but, oh how I hate these cigarettes.

Day 72

Mantra

Say this every time I light up…

I hate smoking so much!

Day 73

Mantra

Getting closer to the end.

What a relief it will be to be free of this horrible addiction.

Day 74

Mantra

Just think, in less than three weeks, I'll never have to smoke these things again.

I really, really want to quit!

Day 75

Mantra

I hate the smell of these things.

Can't wait to quit.

Day 76

Mantra

Made it to another weekend…
On Monday, I'll only have
two weeks to go!!
Boy, I hate these things so much!

Day 77

Mantra

Eleven weeks down!!!
ONLY TWO TO GO!!
I will be so happy when
I finally quit this disgusting habit!

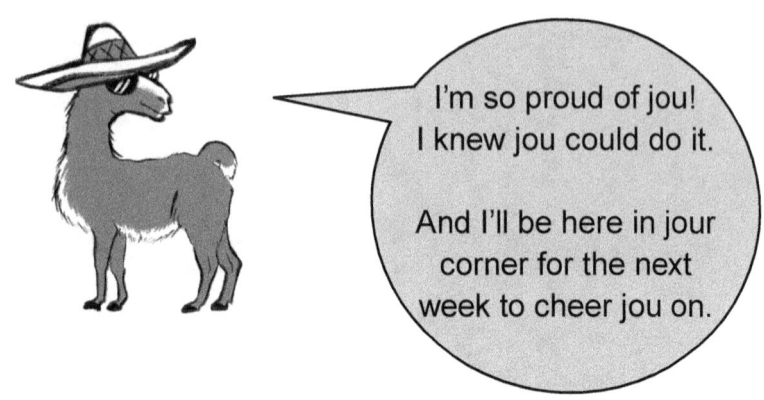

I'm so proud of jou!
I knew jou could do it.

And I'll be here in jour
corner for the next
week to cheer jou on.

Be sure to tell all jour
friends just what jou have
accomplished when jou quit.

Jou can be justly proud of
what jou have done.

I bet jou will be an
inspiration to everyone.

OK, let's get going!

Day 78

Mantra

OK, only fourteen days to go! Wow, I can quit this awful habit in just two weeks.

Day 79

Mantra

Oh, how happy I'm gonna be
when I finally quit smoking...
in less than two weeks.
I can hardly wait.

Day 80

Mantra

Gotta keep smoking…

as much as I always have. Boy, do I ever hate these things.

Day 81

Mantra

This is really hard. I want to quit but I've gotta keep smoking for another week and a half.

Day 82

Mantra

To keep smoking is hard…

To quit will be easy.

Day 83

Mantra

Another weekend is here…

I'm getting close to finally being able to quit. Can't wait!!

Day 84

Mantra

Finally, only one more week to go. I'm going to be so happy to quit.

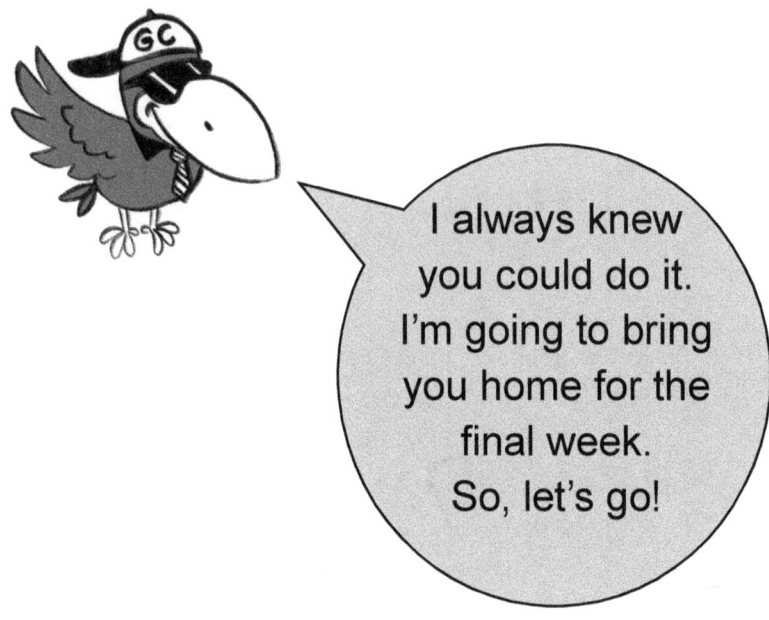

Wow, this has been quite
a journey, hasn't it?
I know that my team and I have
been a burr under your saddle
for the last twelve weeks.
We were doing it for you…

but you've been the strong one
and done all the heavy lifting.

Day 85

Mantra

This is it. My final week… only seven days to go and then I can finally quit these awful cigarettes.

Day 86

Mantra

Why don't I quit right now…
I sure feel like it!

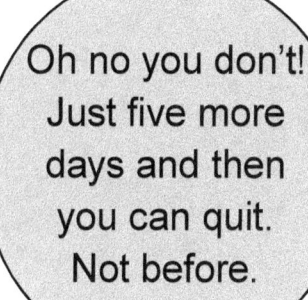
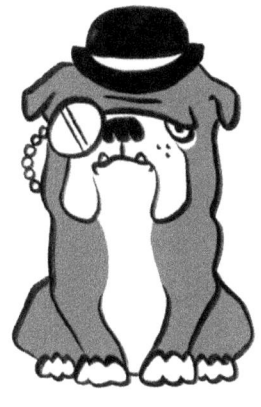

Oh no you don't! Just five more days and then you can quit. Not before.

Sorry to be such a pain, but you know what my job is… I'm the reinforcer, remember? The whole gang is standing by to welcome you at the finish line. You've just about done it, my friend.

Day 87

Mantra

This is great... I've got a whole cheering section to help.

Thanks, guys.

I'll keep smoking like always for another five days, even though I hate it.

Day 88

Mantra

This is the hardest part yet: having to keep smoking when I hate it so much.

Day 89

Mantra

Oh boy... three days to go.
I can hardly wait to throw away
all these stupid, awful cigarettes.

Day 90

Mantra

The second last day….
Yahoo!!
I hate these things, but for one more day I'll keep smoking.

Day 91

Mantra

This is it!
Tonight, I will stop smoking…
Forever!!!!

Never been so happy in my life. Thanks GC, BD, DL, and Toni. You're the best thing that ever happened to me.

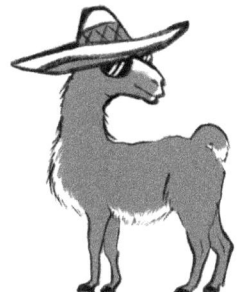
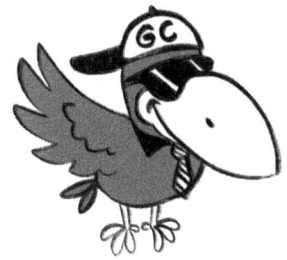

From all of us…
Congratulations!
You did it!
You should be very proud of yourself.
This is the start of a whole new phase of your life.
You will be amazed at all the new sensations you're going to discover.

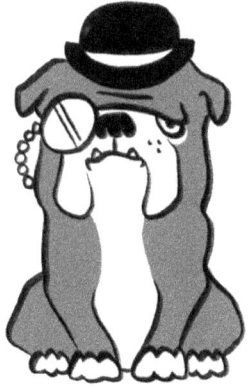
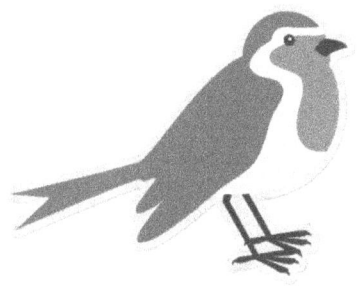

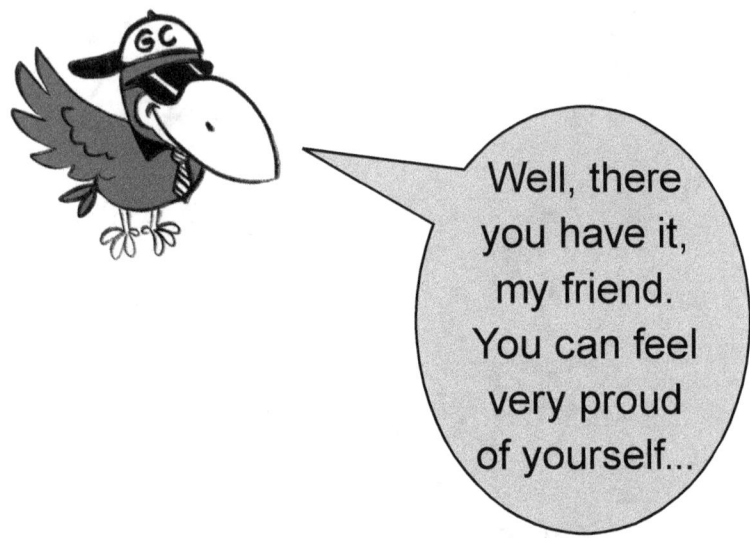

Well, there you have it, my friend. You can feel very proud of yourself...

...You started this journey ninety days ago... three months… and you made it! You stuck it out and put up with my nagging… With BD, DL, and Toni's help and your own determination, you took charge and made a real change in your life. I promise you'll never regret it! Well done! Well done!

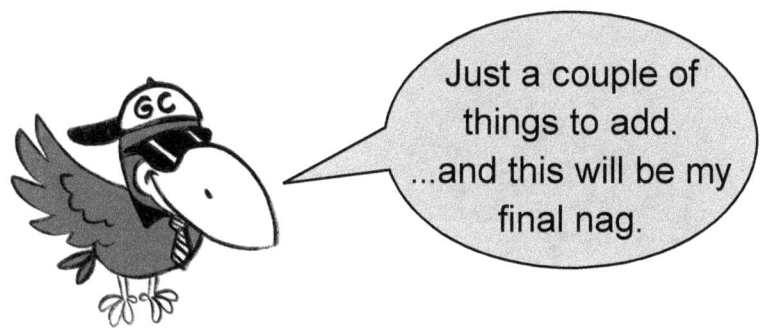

Probably the first thing you'll notice is that food will start to taste really good.

You gotta watch it, though… you may start to eat more 'cause it tastes so much better. You know what that can mean.

Yup... you could start to gain weight.

No big deal. You'll have more energy so you'll be able to burn it off more easily.

We'd all like to know how you're doing, so please give us an update from time to time.

It's been a privilege to help you on your journey. Good luck from all of us.

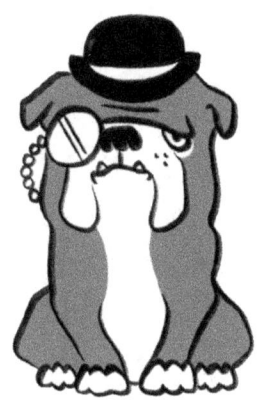

"Hey, GC... we did good, didn't we.

I can't wait for our next adventure."

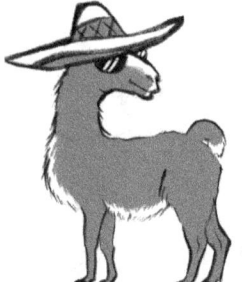

"Jes, me too.

...and wherever we go, jou can yust hop on my back and I'll carry jou all anywhere. After all, that's what I am... a pack animal."

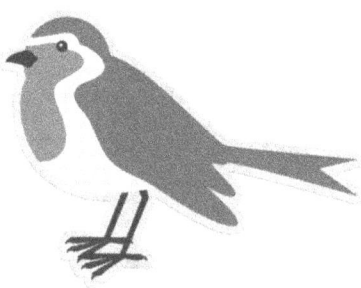

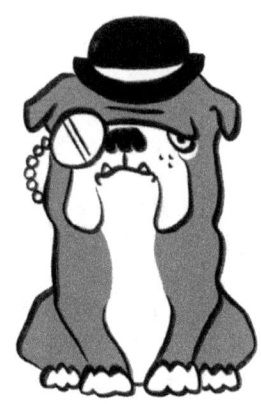
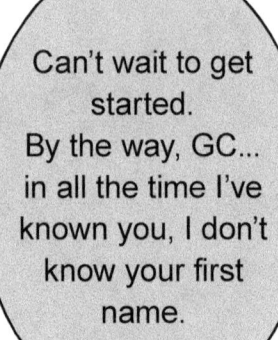

Well, guys, this has been a very rewarding experience for me and I hope for you too. Here's another mantra for all of you… and for our readers as well.

"Success is merely a product of focus.

Focus comes from having a purpose.

Having a purpose comes from being needed.

Being needed comes from serving others."

That's what makes this whole adventure worthwhile — the hope that we've served others… well.

And we'll keep this at the top of our mind as we embark on our newest adventure…

"Do Something Amazing."

Hope to see you all again, next year.

Cheers,

GC

PF Barry – Bio

As someone once opined, "There's a book inside of just about everyone."

Paul Barry took this to heart and decided to see if it were true. Low and behold, *Smokebreaker* was born.

A committed hedonist all his life, the pursuit of happiness has indeed been his life's work. But early on he realized that happiness comes from more than just a bacchanalian focus; it also comes from an inner desire to seek some kind of fulfillment…and that fulfillment, to have meaning, must come from having a purpose which, in turn, comes from being needed. Being needed comes from serving others. From the example set by his father, he has tried to follow that path.

In addition to his father, another important inspiration came from his high school English teacher at Sir Adam Beck Collegiate in London, Ontario.

"Mr. Langford instilled a love of the English language in all his students and for that, I'll be forever grateful," says Mr. Barry.

Having spent most of his career in the public relations and special promotions field, he continues to dabble in some facet of that profession in retirement. In fact, he says, "No one really retires from this profession."

Each life benchmark denotes not the end of a period of one's life; rather, it marks the beginning of a new chapter... most notably expressed upon graduation.

That's why it's called commencement. And another book is already underway... could *Smokebreaker* be the start of a whole new career?

Well, why not?

www.ingramcontent.com/pod-product-compliance
Lightning Source LLC
LaVergne TN
LVHW011715060526
838200LV00051B/2910